Essential Oils for Congestion

Essential Oil Recipes for
Congestion
for Diffusers, Roller Bottles,
Inhalers & more.

Rica V. Gadi

This book is dedicated to all the strong people who are taking responsibility of your own well being and doing something to be better.

All my heartfelt gratitude to the following people: my mom Ruby Jane, you have made me everything I am today; my dad Nestor-- my eternal, my angel, and the source of my perseverance; Mommyling, my spiritual guide ; Ria & Joe, the true witnesses of my transformation and my foundation pillars; Ellie Jane, the sparkle of our eyes;

Juan, thanks for always encouraging me to push harder - you are my ONE; Rocco & Radha, my reason for everything.

The Love of my family and friends is the fountain of inspiration that never runs dry. Thank you for constantly inspiring me, motivating me, and loving me unconditionally.

This book will never be complete without the help of my trusted and talented friends the #NOWsuperstars and my #oilbularya friends

Blending Essential Oils to use for a ver
specific reason has become very popular i
the recent years. There are several reasor
why this is so. Blending EOs is basical
about inhaling - as it has been proven tha
aromas have the ability to trigger feeling
emotions and personal memories.

With this in mind, it is obvious that everyon
is unique when it comes to what trigger
your senses. It all boils down to person
preference for the aroma to trigger wha
you want to unleash. Everyone is differer
and we all connect to the aroma differentl
so what might work for one might not wor
for another person.

Of course, we also want the blend w
personalize to be therapeutic. This is th
best reason why to blend essential oils. W
want the blend we create to help us with
very specific emotion or physical conditio
As much as smelling good is important in
blend, it is more important that we blen
oils that is not only pleasing to the smell bu
also produces the therapeutic effect we ar
after.

Then you have to think abou
contraindications. Making sure the blen
you create is safe to use.

I suggest that before blending find out if the oils you are using is safe for a condition you may have example, if you are pregnant, or have specific allergies. Consult your physician prior to moving forward.

The recipes I have in this book is a compilation of what has proven to work and favored by hundreds of EO enthusiasts. It takes out the guesswork to get you started.

Again, we urge you to read the recipes and make sure that this is safe for you to try.

The book is very specific to a physical and emotional condition. There are several recipes here because you might want to rotate and you may like one and not the other. There is also a variety of application. Some of us prefer to diffuse, some to make roller bottles, and others to create sprays.

I hope you enjoy this compilation, feel free to use the notes section and jot down your fave blends. There is a wonderful world of EO blending - this is just the beginning.

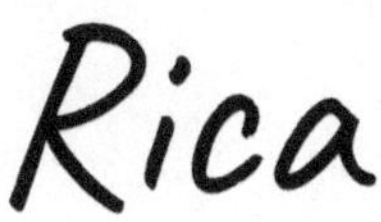

Congestions are usually caused by a number of things like seasonal allergies, weather change, and/ or viruses. Contributing factors for causing a congestion could also be the flu or a common cold. Congestions are not only physically annoying but causes irritation in your lungs, which usually causes coughing, which could elevate a common cold into an infection.

Persistent congestion could be caused by a number of things like a long-term respiratory tract infection, like chronic bronchitis. Post Nasal Drip – caused by mucus trickling down your throat from the back of the nose, usually stemming from rhinitis or sinusitis.

Usually EOs don't cure the congestion, what it does is assist in taming the symptoms that are connected to it, the common cold and seasonal allergies. Essential Oils help relieve congestion by soothing the throat, combating bacteria, and controlling inflammation.

It could aid to clear your lungs and help fast-track the healing process, making them amazing for dealing with the symptoms.

Why use Essential oils for congestion ar
how can it help?

Viruses are seasonal and at any point in th
year it becomes rampant and could caus
Congestion. EOs help in combating thes
illnesses and fight allergies. it als
strengthens your immune system. In th
event you have already been stricken, the
can assist in healing faster. The versatility
EOs allows us to use it in many differer
ways and apply in a variety of ways, giving u
multiple options for intervention that be
help in healing symptoms or the illne
itself.

Since most congestion and other respirato
issues are usually caused by viruse
Essential oils' antiviral properties can k
great in actually preventing a congestic
before it even starts to happen.

Table of Contents

ESSENTIAL OILS FOR CONGESTION

Some mild respiratory ailments such as cough or cold are viewed to be inevitable in a sense. They can happen to you sometime of the year even if you tried your best in boosting your immune system. At times that these ailments remain untreated, some complications can happen which can affect our rest and sleep. Congestion for example, is one of the effects of having cough or cold as our air passage is blocked or clogged. This will result to difficulty in breathing, and heck even disturbs you from your sweet slumber. So, it is very important to know what are the possible remedies that we can have in reducing congestion for our own comfort. As there are a plethora of medicines that you can buy in pharmacies and drugstores, you can also be treated by oils, not just ordinary oils; but pure essential oils. If this is your first time hearing about it, take a read as we list down below the most suggested essential oils for congestion.

Eucalyptus

Eucalyptus is recognized for its ability to treat respiratory ailments such as cough. In the late 70's, it was used to treat symptoms relating to bronchial and chest issues. Eucalyptus contains a substance called eucalyptil which has a spicy yet cooling effect. This compound possesses antimicrobial, antiviral, and antibacterial properties which work together to open clogged airways, reduce the frequency of cough, impede propagation of phlegm and mucus, and most importantly relieve congestion.

For inhalation process, add 10-15 drops of eucalyptus essential oil to a bowl of boiling water. Just simply breathe in the vaporized soothing scent for at least 5-10 minutes while it tries to calm and clear you nasal cavity.

You may also try to mix a drop of eucalyptus oil and
drops of lavender oil in cup of hot water, dampen
washcloth in the mixture and directly apply to you
forehead as the lavender oil can also calm your body an
mind. If used topically, you may combine it with olive
jojoba oil and apply to the chest as vapor rub to reduc
congestion.

Thyme

Thyme is one of the most effective antioxidants in th
planet that serves as an aid for respiratory, immune, ar
nervous system. It also contains antispasmodi
antibacterial, and antiseptic properties which is ve
useful in treating sinus congestion and pressure.

Thyme as one of the essential oils for congestion is be
used through topical application. Have your ow
mixture of 1:1 ratio with a carrier oil for best results.

Lemon

From a bright fruit which we can usually have a taste
in some dishes and drinks, who has an idea that lemo
can work as an essential oil for congestion too? Lemon
fairly styptic and is a known remedy for sinus problem
Lemon has high levels of citric acid and Vitamin C so
fights off toxins and germs which then eliminate th
bacteria that may lead to infection. Lemon can be use
as well in boosting the immune system and decrea.
the occurrence of respiratory ailments. Aside from tha
it is most effective in breaking down the mucus an
releasing it to reduce/relieve congestion.

When you feel that sinus pressure or congestion star
rub 2-5 drops of lemon essential oil and directly apply
neck or chest. Repeat this process as necessary as it ge

during the day. Since lemon is proven to be safe for ingestion, it is also great to have a cup of tea with a few drops of the oil mixed with a taste of honey. This will also help relieve congestion and sore throat.

Peppermint

Because of peppermint's antibacterial and antiviral properties, it is considered as one of the most effective essential oils for cough and cold. This herb contains menthol which is best known for the relief it gives for congestion so it improves your nasal airflow by unclogging your sinuses. Menthol also offers a cooling sensation which soothes your sore and scratchy throat. But it will still be the mild sedative and potent properties it have which makes it a remedy for sinus congestion and pressure.

You may enjoy these peppermint oil benefits in several ways. Have 3-5 drops of peppermint essential oil in a diffuser as it disperses the vaporized soothing scent as it clears your air passage. You can also topically apply 2-3 drops of the oil to the back of your neck and temples, and chest. If you want to create your own vapor rub, try to mix this oil with eucalyptus essential oil for a more satisfying experience. An important note to observe, do not apply near your eyes as it causes irritation.

Clove

Clove made it to the list for being one of the top essential oils for congestion. Just like with the other oils, clove also contains antiseptic and antibacterial properties which help in alleviating the sinus congestion.

You can use clove oil in several ways and we will discu
some of them. Through diffusion, have a genero
amount of drops of the oil in your diffuser for at least
minutes. The passive anti-inflammatory property effe
will slacken your air passage, which helps redu
congestion and other respiratory problems. You m
also try to rub the oil into your chest or bridge of t
nose to improve breathing and open air passage. Y
may also try to add 3-4 drops of clove oil to a glass
warm water. This can prevent other respiratory ailmer
and infections.

I know you would not like to be disturbed from yc
deep sleep just because of difficulty in breathing caus
by congestion. So, it is necessary to have a faster rel
from this discomfort to continuously drift into yc
slumber. As the benefits were discussed, you can ta
advantage of these essential oils for congestion ma
for you when you need them the most. However, it
important to note that you can't take essential c
without knowing their properties because there mig
be allergic reactions.

It is also worth mentioning that the following oils a
worth checking out for Congestion : **Tea Tree, Oregar
Cinnamon, Cedarwood, Ginger, Lavender a
Rosemary**

The Blending Process

These EOs are categorized by aromas, and EOs from the same group usually blend fantastically together.

- Floral – Lavender, Geranium, Jasmine
- Woodsy – Pine, Cedarwood
- Earthy – Vetiver, Patchouli
- Herbaceous – Marjoram, Rosemary, Basil
- Minty – Peppermint, Spearmint, Wintergreen
- Medicinal – Eucalyptus, Frankincense, Melaleuca
- Spicy – Pepper, Clove, Cinnamon
- Oriental – Ginger, Patchouli
- Citrus – Wild Orange, Lemon, Lime

Select oils that will give you with the health benefits you are looking to remedy. For increased energy choose: Grapefruit, Lemon, Orange, or Citrus. For Calming and Relaxation choose: Lavender, Cedarwood, or Chamomile. You are encouraged to experiment and play with your oils to see which blends work for you.

TIPS:

- Combine Floral EOs with Woodsy, Spicy and Citrus aromas
- Minty EOs with Woodsy, Earthy, Herbaceous and Citrus aromas
- Earthy EOs with Woodsy and Minty aromas
- Citrus EOs with Floral, Woodsy, Minty, Spicy and Oriental aromas

Diffuse

Diffusing Essential Oils is the safest method to enjoy Essential Oils without the risk of an allergic reaction.

Diffusing Essential Oils
Some Tidbits You Need To Know

Our sense of smell is one of our most powerful sense
and as you have noticed in your own experience th
some scents affect your more positively in your minc
than others. The body contains over 1,000 recepto
for smell—way more receptors than for any of ot
other senses.

Diffusion Essential Oils means the process vaporiz
oils into air by releasing tiny amounts into the a
Inhalation is totally safe and is super low risk. Chanc
of any EO rising to dangerous levels while diffusion
slim to none.

Diffusing Essential Oils around newborns, babie
young children, pregnant or nursing women, ar
pets should be done with caution. Read up on safety

It is advisable that Diffusing Essential Oils for on
about 15-30 minutes at a time to be most effectiv
NEVER leave your diffuser on overnight. Make su
your diffuser is filled with the right amount of wat
and you understand the operating directions.

While diffusing essential oils, be sure that your spac
has great ventilation. Crack a window open if th
scent become to strong.

Never add Carrier Oils to your diffuser. This may caus
your diffuser to malfunction. Clean your diffuser
least 3 times a week with warm water and natur
soap to ensure the diffuser is well maintained ar
bacteria and mold does not accumulate.

Diffusing Essential Oils
Basic Guidelines

Just a few things you need to know and prepare before getting started Diffusing Essential Oils.

Things you need:
Ultrasonic Oil Diffuser
Essential Oils
Water

Just follow the number of drops in the recipe, drop on to an oil diffuser and fill the rest with water.

All diffusers are different and will have its own water minimum and maximum level. Read the diffuser instruction before use.

Ideally, it is best to diffuse for 15-30 minutes and turn off the diffuser. The effect should be good for at least 2-3 hours. Turn your diffuser back on after 3 hours to reinforce oil diffusing effects.

It is not advisable to use EO in humidifiers.

These are not made to release EOS

Diffuser Recipes

Here's a thought for you:

You may be wondering how aroma can simp
eliminate symptoms. There's a simple answer to thi
Aroma is simply a by-product of diffusing. It's th
added benefit but in reality the real benefit com
from the air we breathe and how the body eas
absorbs the essential oils released in the air. It works
ways, not only does it improve the air quality yc
breath by disinfecting and eliminating pollutants
also allows your glands to absorb the healir
elements of the EOs released in the air molecules,

So for here are a few recipes that can help yc
manage symptoms and actual issues regarding th
matter :

3 Drops Lemon
3 Drops Scotch Pine
3 Drops Lavender
1 Drop Peppermint

----

3 Drops Juniper Berry
4 Drops Rosemary
4 Drops Frankincense

----

4 Drops Cypress
6 Drops Grapefruit

----

5 Drops Cedarwood
4 Drops Lavender
1 Drop Chamomile
1 Drop Eucalyptus (optional)

5-7 Drops Pine or Cedarwood
5-7 Drops Lavender
4 Drops Eucalyptus
1 Drop Lemon

3-5 Drops Rosemary
2 Drops Thyme
1 Drop Peppermint

----

3 Drops Peppermint
3 Drops Lemon
3 Drops Eucalyptus

----

2 Drops Oregano
2 Drops Tea Tree
2 Drops Peppermint
2 Drops Lavender
2 Drops Lemon

3 Drops Tea Tree
2 Drops Lavender
2 Drops Peppermint

----

4 Drops Lavender
4 Drops Peppermint
2 Drops Frankincense
2 Drops Basil

----

3 Drops Rosemary
2 Drops Eucalyptus
2 Drops Peppermint
1 Drops Cypress
1 Drops Lemon

----

2 Drops Lemon
1 Drops Lime
2 Drops Peppermint
1 Drops Rosemary
2 Drops Eucalyptus
1 Drop Clove

----

3 Drops RC
3 Drops Lemon
3 Drops Purification

----

2 Drops Eucalyptus
1 Drops Peppermint